POWERFUL QUESTIONS TO HELP YOU MOVE FORWARD IN YOUR LIFE

"What you are afraid to do is a clear indicator of the next thing you need to do."
—ANONYMOUS

BY MICHAEL GARLIN

Everyday Is Monday Publications

ISBN: 1496091914

ISBN 13: 9781496091918

Library of Congress Control Number: 2014904087

CreateSpace Independent Publishing Platform

North Charleston, South Carolina

ACKNOWLEDGMENTS

To the love of my life, Mindy; the greatest guy and son ever, Brad; the most beautiful daughter, Marisa; my life coach, Mary Beth, for helping me move forward in my life; my mother who, like any mother, lets me know how much she loves me; and all of my relatives, friends, and colleagues who have always been my support over the years. A very special thank you to my new friend Eugene, who encouraged me to publish my book.

DEDICATION

In memory of my father, Gene Garlin, who was and will always be my best friend.

Please read page by page and create your own passions, dreams, and desires to each powerful question. The biggest question to ask yourself is: Am I ready to live a healthy life?

"My suggestion is to go out and purchase a really nice pen. There is something about a good pen that gives the confidence to write something special." –GENE A. GARLIN

A LETTER FROM ME TO YOU

Dear reader,

I have one very important question to ask you prior to you delving into this book: Are you ready to live a healthy and truthful life? I spent most of my life being untruthful to myself. Why is it that I always failed on diets? Unless we are truly committed to being healthy, these weight-loss programs just won't work.

You can go on any diet and lose weight. However, you need to realize that it's not about weight loss. It's completely about getting healthy.

In April 2013 I was told that my type 2 diabetes was now on the cusp of becoming type 1. "What can I do to get healthy?" My doctor explained, "Michael, you need to get thin, you need to remove the fat, and you need to get healthy."

It was now or never. I needed to take care of myself. I needed to eat real food. I needed to take care of me. Was I ready to live a healthy life? My answer was *yes*. Why? Why would I lead a life of being unhealthy? This just didn't make sense anymore. It was time to feel great, climb a mountain, swim across a lake, and most of all, change my outlook on what I really wanted in life. I knew that the power to finally make the changes I needed was possible. I had to understand why I did what I did and what I needed to do to make the necessary changes.

This book provides you with powerful questions that will help you make changes in all aspects of your life. Your career, your personal relationships—really, every aspect of your life. The investment of a few hours, maybe a few weeks, possibly a few months to really consider the questions that are being asked of you.

After a lifetime of feeling unhealthy I finally dropped sixty-plus pounds and reversed my diabetes completely. I have changed careers to fit my goals and dreams. I am closer with my family than ever before. The bonus is that I went from a 44 waist pant to a thirty-four waist pant, I exercise daily, and my blood work is crazy great.

I am now completely convinced that we are what we eat. Living a life that is true to yourself is the only way to live. I have chosen to live eating a whole-foods, plant-based diet. I cured every one of my ailments by eating real food. The greatest gift you can give yourself is the gift of health, and it's all in your control.

Enjoy reading, and definitely get yourself a good pen (great advice from my dad) to answer these life changing questions. Your answers will lead you down your own personal path of living the life you have chosen. Again I ask myself everyday: Am I ready to live a healthy and truthful life?

Michael Garlin

Michael's Three Rules for Completing this Book

1. Think through each question, and answer it with true honesty. If you are not true to yourself, how can you expect to move forward in your life?

2. Ask for help. If you are stuck, go to the people who care about you the most and ask them to give insight. This was eye-opening for me. Dig deep because this will truly help you accomplish the answers you are seeking.

3. Answer every question completely. You may find yourself changing careers, succeeding in school, building new and long-lasting relationships, and living the dreams you were meant to live. Most of all, you will start getting healthy, both mentally and physically.

That's it. Enjoy the book, and if you get stuck, drop me an e-mail at michael@iamstartingonmonday.com. I will do my best to get back to you as quickly as possible.

How do I define **achievement**?

Read, study hard, and make time for yourself, and you will reap the rewards. There is no success without pain, without difficulty, without negatives, without overcoming obstacles, without conflict. I have never had true achievement or pleasure without enduring some type of pain; it's just not possible. However, the outcomes of achievement far outweigh the pain.

"There are no gains without pains." –BENJAMIN FRANKLIN

What does the word **achievement** mean to you?

What have been your top five achievements in your life?

What do you still want to achieve?

What are you willing to give up?

POWERFUL QUESTIONS TO HELP YOU MOVE FORWARD IN YOUR LIFE

What does **attitude** mean to me?

I have always had a positive attitude toward life and work. Circumstances arise that are usually out of my control, but I realize that it's how I react to these circumstances that determines my attitude. I have found that a poor attitude usually contributes to failure. You can fail with a positive attitude as well; however, a positive attitude seems to lessen the blow.

"There are two big forces at work, external and internal. We have very little control over external forces such as tornados, earthquakes, floods, disasters, illness, and pain. What really matters is the internal force. How do I respond to those disasters? Over that I have complete control." –LEO BUSCAGLIA

POWERFUL QUESTIONS TO HELP YOU
MOVE FORWARD IN YOUR LIFE

What is your **attitude** today?

What is it about attitude that is important to you?

What are the external forces that keep knocking you down?

What attitude are you going to choose?

POWERFUL QUESTIONS TO HELP YOU
MOVE FORWARD IN YOUR LIFE

What do I need in life to stay true to my **beliefs**?

I know I will be successful in whatever I set out to accomplish. That is what I truly believe. My desire and persistence control my beliefs. I will get there!

I realize that I will always be on the road to happiness. I always have to remember to go into situations with my eyes wide open and with my beliefs in check to truly seize the opportunities in front of me.

"Whether you think you can or think you can't—you are right."
–HENRY FORD

POWERFUL QUESTIONS TO HELP YOU MOVE FORWARD IN YOUR LIFE

What do you need in life to stay true to your **beliefs**?

What if you do stay true to your beliefs, and what if you don't?

POWERFUL QUESTIONS TO HELP YOU
MOVE FORWARD IN YOUR LIFE

What do you think it is difficult to make the **right choice**?

We all have the power to make our own choices. No one should make our choices for us. Intuition and thought-out perspectives have always guided me in my decision-making process. Surrounding myself with the right positive force (people) allows me to make the right choices. Learning how to look at the glass as overflowing and understanding how to look at different perspectives allows me to choose the right path.

"You don't have to buy from anyone. You don't have to work at any particular job. You don't have to participate in any given relationship. You can choose." –HARRY BROWNE

What are your **choices**?

What guides you in making tough choices? Have you ever really thought about how and when you decide? Start documenting how you make choices, and think if there are other ways you can make those decisions.

POWERFUL QUESTIONS TO HELP YOU MOVE FORWARD IN YOUR LIFE

What **circumstance** has control over me?

Circumstances are out of my control; it's how I manage these circumstances that makes me tough. This is truly where I either move forward in life or let outside influences drag me down. I am only in control of my response to the circumstance. I am a firm believer that you can change your circumstance.

"What's going on in the inside shows on the outside."
–EARL NIGHTINGALE

POWERFUL QUESTIONS TO HELP YOU
MOVE FORWARD IN YOUR LIFE

What **circumstances** are controlling you?

What is holding you back? What can you do to change your circumstances?

POWERFUL QUESTIONS TO HELP YOU
MOVE FORWARD IN YOUR LIFE

What am I worth? What **compensation** do I deserve for my efforts?

I really want to be compensated for my hard work. It is very painful to put in your blood, sweat, and tears and not receive the proper payment for the output. Payment doesn't always equal money; sometimes payment is recognition. Everyone needs to be compensated in some way.

"For everything you have missed, you have gained something else; and for everything you gain, you lose something else"
–RALPH WALDO EMERSON

What are you worth? What is your **compensation**?

What is your desired outcome for the time you put into your career, relationships, or body?

POWERFUL QUESTIONS TO HELP YOU
MOVE FORWARD IN YOUR LIFE

What do I need to do to build up my **confidence**?

Confidence is all about preparation. Study, do the research, practice the presentation, and than do it all over again. Can you climb a mountain without preparing? Can you take an exam without studying? Can you learn to walk without falling down? Can you become healthy without eating healthy?

Practice, practice, practice, practice, practice, practice.

Now I'm confident. I have failed over and over and over again until I finally got it right. If that doesn't build confidence, nothing does.

"Confidence doesn't come out of nowhere. It's a result of something...hours and days and weeks and years of constant work and dedication." –ROGER STAUBACH

Be prepared! –BOY SCOUT MOTTO

POWERFUL QUESTIONS TO HELP YOU
MOVE FORWARD IN YOUR LIFE

What does **confidence** mean to you?

How do you build your confidence? The real question is, what is
your desired outcome?

How do I deal with **conflict**?

Early in my life and career, I avoided conflicts at school, at work, with supervisors, with my spouse, with my children, with everyone. Avoiding conflict was actually making me ill. I sometimes felt taken advantage of and that I had no control over most situations.

I finally changed. I had no choice. Wow, do I feel better for it. I meet conflict head on now. There is no other way.

"When confronted with a conflict, listen to what the other person has to say without interrupting and without emotions to the best of your ability. I know that there may be times to walk away. However, with a calm demeanor, conflicts can be resolved quickly, honestly, and with good intentions." –MINDY GARLIN

"When we direct our thoughts properly, we can control our emotions." –W. CLEMENT STONE

How do you deal with **conflict**?

What continually seems to be the main obstacle? If you can't manage the conflict and it fails, what will you do? How do you manage conflicts?

POWERFUL QUESTIONS TO HELP YOU MOVE FORWARD IN YOUR LIFE

What do I need to do to stay in **control** of my own success?

"Who's in control?" "I am in control."

It has taken me years to truly understand that only I have control over myself. I have no control over anyone but myself. Repeat: I have no control over anyone except myself.

When we control our decisions, we control our actions, and this is the path to our success.

"When you take charge of your life, there is no longer a need to ask permission of other people or society at large....When you ask permission, you give someone veto power over your life."
–GEOFFREY F. ABERT

Who and what **controls** your success?

Are you truly in control? If not, why?

What does **courage** mean to me?

Courage means getting up in the morning and facing the day with honor, truthfulness, and a sense of pride. That, to me, is true courage.

"Courage is to confront fear, resistance, outside forces, and misfortunes, and knowing that it's OK to be afraid." —ANONYMOUS

POWERFUL QUESTIONS TO HELP YOU MOVE FORWARD IN YOUR LIFE

What does **courage** mean to you?

POWERFUL QUESTIONS TO HELP YOU MOVE FORWARD IN YOUR LIFE

What is my true **desire**?

Desire is the power to succeed. Without desire, why are we here?

My desires are my commitments to myself, to my heart, and to my life. I have many desires, and to achieve them I must be ready to commit to them. Write them down. Read them every night. Be persistent in following your desires.

"Always bear in mind that your own resolution to succeed is more important than any other one thing." –ABRAHAM LINCOLN

What are your true **desires**?

Write them down. Read them, live them, and honor them. This is your road to happiness!

What do I **enjoy** in life?

I always enjoy the little things and sharing those little things with the people I love.

I am now an author, a business owner, and a motivational speaker. I am a healthy man who enjoys walking, talking, and being my true self. I am enjoying life as it was meant to be.

I definitely have days when I want to stay in bed, but that is usually because I went to bed too late.

"I'd rather be a failure in something that I love than a success in something that I don't." –GEORGE BURNS

What do you **enjoy** in life?

Write it down and start living it.

What is my **environment** like at home and work?

Surround yourself in a place that feels right. When you wake up and get ready for the day, how do you feel? Look around. Do you enjoy where you are when starting your day? When you get to work, what does it feel like to sit in your chair, your car, or wherever you start your day? Does it feel right?

I try to create an environment that motivates me and puts a smile on my face. If it's messy, clean it up. Put pictures up that inspire you. What else do you need?

I can't find who stated, "Home is where the heart is," but that is the truth.

What does your **environment** feel like?

What can you change to make your environment a good one? It is better to work somewhere inspiring. Sometimes just adding a lamp changes everything.

POWERFUL QUESTIONS TO HELP YOU MOVE FORWARD IN YOUR LIFE

What does **excellence** mean to me?

To me, excellence means crossing the T's, dotting the I's, and knowing that I gave it my all. Doing well with the little things makes something excellent. Quality over quantity; that is excellence.

"It is just the little difference between the good and the best that makes the difference between the artist and the artisan. It is just the little touches after the average man would quit that make the master's fame." –ORISON SWETT MARDEN

What does **excellence** mean for you?

POWERFUL QUESTIONS TO HELP YOU
MOVE FORWARD IN YOUR LIFE

What does **failure** mean to me?

Without failure, there are no successes. How can you learn without failing? Admit when you fail because you will only win when you aren't afraid to lose. You must accept who you are, because you are, and that will always be the beginning, the middle, and the end on your road to success. Don't ever apologize for your failure, because you should have no regrets. Learn from your failures and move on.

My father gave me a greeting card one day when I was stressing over a failure. It read:

"Finish each day and be done with it. You have done what you could. Some blunders and absurdities have crept in; forget them as soon as you can. Tomorrow is a new day. You shall begin it serenely and with too high a spirit to be encumbered with your old nonsense."
–RALPH WALDO EMERSON

POWERFUL QUESTIONS TO HELP YOU
MOVE FORWARD IN YOUR LIFE

What does the word **failure** mean to you?

Do you own up to your failures? Post the Emerson quote from above wherever you work—at your car, your desk, etc.—and always read it before you go home.

Faith is only something you believe, not something that can be given to you by someone else. It's something I will always continue to seek out.

Take classes, listen to lectures, read books, and most of all, have a child—and if you can't, get a puppy. The birth of a child will give you the faith you need to move forward in life.

"The fact that I can plant a seed and it becomes a flower, share a bit of knowledge and it becomes another's, smile at someone and receive a smile in return are to me continual spiritual exercises."
–LEO BUSCAGLIA

"Who has seen the wind?" –CHRISTINA ROSSETTI

POWERFUL QUESTIONS TO HELP YOU
MOVE FORWARD IN YOUR LIFE

Faith. No question here. Just something to think about, something to write about. How about a poem? What is inside of you?

What does **fear** do to me?

How do I face fear?
Fear sometimes handcuffs me, makes me ill, or just gives me that feeling in my throat that I can't breathe.

I take comfort in knowing that there is freedom at the other end of fear. Conquering your fear will give you the confidence to succeed. I am always ready to get out of my comfort zone.

This is my personal mantra when I coach someone. My good friend Tatiana sent this to me because she felt that it personifies my inner spirit.

"Come to the edge," he said.
They said, "We are afraid."
"Come to the edge," he said.
They came.
He pushed them…and they flew.
–GUILLAUME APOLLINAIRE

How do you handle **fear**?

Where do you feel it on your body? Everyone is afraid of something. What are you afraid of? The harder question is, how will you face your fear in the future?

What am I willing to give up for **freedom**?

Freedom has wings. Freedom has laughter. Freedom brings new experiences to all of us each and every day. With freedom, there are sacrifices and a price to pay.

I think of my monthly "dads night out poker night." This is the ultimate freedom. However, I have to sacrifice by doing a lot of household chores the next day. The freedom to write this book brings the sacrifice of not spending time with my children or not sleeping.

There is always risk with freedom. I am a firm believer of taking some risk each and every day.

"I know but one freedom, and that is the freedom of the mind."
–ANTOINE DE SAINT-EXUPERY

POWERFUL QUESTIONS TO HELP YOU
MOVE FORWARD IN YOUR LIFE

What is your **freedom**?

What do you sacrifice for your freedom?

What **fulfills** me?

Fulfillment—this is what makes me tick. My fulfillment comes from my heart. Living from my heart each and every day to the best of my ability brings me fulfillment.

My personal and most important heart full words that fulfill me each day:

Family, charity, humor, synergy, creativity, dependability, flex-ibility, friendliness, happiness, heart, intuitiveness, warmth, truth, gratitude, making a difference!

"The only wealth is life." –HENRY DAVID THOREAU

"You have succeeded in life when all you really want is only what you really need." –VERNON HOWARD

POWERFUL QUESTIONS TO HELP YOU MOVE FORWARD IN YOUR LIFE

What are your heart full words that create your **fulfillment**?

Take a day to write them down. What makes you tick?

What does **giving** mean to me?

Giving is the key to getting! However, don't expect to get; just appreciate it when it comes and say thank you.

Start networking with your friends, family or aquaintances. Give them what they need to help them in whatever they are searching for at that moment in their life. I find this to be monumental in their lives and for some reason for my life as well. It is an incredible feeling when you can help someone when they are stuck.

I asked my daughter, Marisa, when she was five what giving meant to her. As we were hugging, she told me that giving me a hug was giving her warmth all over. What's better than that?

"What you keep to yourself, you lose. What you give away, you keep forever." –UNKNOWN

How do you **give**?

What does giving mean to you?

What are my personal **goals**?

The purpose behind a personal goal is to create a vision of accomplishment. Five steps in creating my goals.

One: Create a vision of your future self.
Two: Set realistic goals based on your vision.
Three: Break the larger goal into smaller, shorter-term goals.
Four: Eliminate what is getting in your way of achieving your goals.
Five: Be accountable to yourself first and then your future.

Example:
One: I visualized what it would feel like to be thin and healthy. I still do this daily.
Two: 261 to 184 pounds; I didn't gain all this weight and get to the cusp of type 1 diabetes in one day.
Three: One to two pounds per week. Slowly remove processed foods, sugar, alcohol, bread, and fat (red meat, chicken, fish and dairy - I guess I am Vegan).
Four: External obstacles was my biggest issue. This included people who told me what and how I should eat; I called them FPs: Food Pushers. Once I eliminated them, yahoo! Although my

mother, Carole, and my mother-in-law, Annette, can be FPs all day long. I love them very much.

Five: - One day at a time. Becoming healthy is a life long task and I realized that to be true to myself I needed to attack this one day at a time.

"The indispensable first step to getting the things you want out of life is this: Decide what you want." –BEN STEIN

What are your **goals**?

What are your visions of accomplishments? Do you have written **goals**? If not, start writing them today, and then read them and live them every day. Pick your biggest vision and set your goals.

How do I want to **grow** as an individual?

The only way to grow is with honor, trust, and passion. The key is to experience life each and every day. Without risk, without knowledge, without doing, we tend to stagnate. Hold your head up and your shoulders back, and walk into your everyday life realizing that you are going to move forward each and every day.

"A man either lives life as it happens to him, meets it head on and licks it, or he turns his back on it and starts to wither away."
–GENE RODDENBERRY

POWERFUL QUESTIONS TO HELP YOU
MOVE FORWARD IN YOUR LIFE

How do you want to **grow** each and every day?

Stand or sit tall when writing this answer. It helps.

What does the word **happiness** mean to me?

When my day is full of learning, growing, accomplishing, and living my passions, this brings happiness.

I know when others are not happy; either they tell you they aren't happy, or they will walk and talk unhappiness. For me, I just don't want to be around unhappy people (who does?). It's like I am running an obstacle course to avoid unhappiness.

I have my unhappy days. This is when I need to read my goals, review my values, or ask someone to tell me a good joke. Have goals—have a lot of goals—read them every day, and live to accomplish as many of them as possible. Also find a good joke. Watch a great comedian on TV. This always makes me happy.

"Happiness is not pleasure. It is victory." –ZIG ZIGLAR

What truly brings you **happiness**?

When you can answer this question without fear, you will live and breathe happiness each and every day moving forward. It is all in your attitude. You have control.

Imagination: Do I ever imagine?

Thank you Walt Disney.

Do you see all your possibilities, everything that can be done with your life and how it can and will be done? I can make it happen. I imagine every day, sometimes every hour, what it would feel like, what it would mean, what I need to do to make my dreams, goals and life complete and fulfilled.

I love imagining winning the lottery. I get in a lot of fights with my wife about how we are going to spend the money.

"A man to carry on a successful business must have imagination. He must think in a vision, a dream of the whole thing."
–CHARLES M. SCHWAB

POWERFUL QUESTIONS TO HELP YOU
MOVE FORWARD IN YOUR LIFE

Do you **imagine**?

If so, what do you imagine? Make it a habit and enjoy your imagination. Using your imagination is very uplifting and can create some pretty incredible things.

Love

A huge question - What does love mean to me?

Everything!

When we have learned to love, we have learned to live. I absolutely love my wife, my daughter, my son, my brother, my friends, my parents, my in-laws, my brothers- and sisters-in-law, my nieces and nephews, my family.

We need to learn to love.

"Love is all you need." –THE BEATLES

"If you have it, you don't need to have anything else, and if you don't have it, it doesn't much matter what else you have."
–SIR JAMES M. BARRIE

Whom do you **love**?

What do you love? How do you learn from love?

POWERFUL QUESTIONS TO HELP YOU MOVE FORWARD IN YOUR LIFE

What concerns me most about **money**?

What is my desired outcome?

I have heard that money is the root of all evil. I have heard that money is freedom. Money to me is a crutch and an excuse for not doing things you truly love. What if I only had more money? I need more money to become successful. Money is your saboteur!

I am the wealthiest man I know. The little things in life make you wealthy, not the green stuff. Take a look at the people you love; they are worth more than anything in your wallet.

Going to sleep every night with my beautiful wife, tucking my daughter into bed, speaking to my son on the phone a few times a week, giving my mother a hug, talking to my brother, spending time with family, feeling the warmth of the sun on my face, watching children play and laugh, watching a good comedy, taking the train into the city each day, walking my dog—this is what truly matters. Worrying about how much money I have is a waste of time. Living life is all that matters.

"Think and grow rich." –NAPOLEON HILL

What does **money** truly mean to you?

What is your desired outcome? Is money holding you back from doing or not doing what you desire, and if so, why?

POWERFUL QUESTIONS TO HELP YOU MOVE FORWARD IN YOUR LIFE

What truly **motivates** me?

We have three choices as individuals: We can decide to do something, we can decide to do nothing, or we can decide not to decide. Being honest with myself every day is my motivation to know what I really want in life. I am always in a position to decide.

Our hearts usually guide us, realizing what we truly want, creating a plan. That is motivation.

"Know thyself." –SOCRATES

POWERFUL QUESTIONS TO HELP YOU
MOVE FORWARD IN YOUR LIFE

What **motivates** you?

What is just one more possibility?

Where do I find my next **opportunity**?

Get out of your house, get out of your office, get out of your cubi-cle, and start meeting people. This is where your next opportu-nity exists. Opportunity is everywhere, and if you search for it, you shall find it.

Today or tomorrow start having breakfast, lunch, dinner, and snacks with everyone you know and everyone you don't know. I meet people on LinkedIn all the time. It's fun to get to know some-one new.

Ask them how they are doing. Ask about them and forget about you. Give to them and you will get back. Don't expect anything back because eventually the whole universe will give back in ways you least expect.

"You must make your own opportunities. It's easy. Just start to learn about the people around you and forget about yourself."
–CHAD COE

POWERFUL QUESTIONS TO HELP YOU
MOVE FORWARD IN YOUR LIFE

Where is your next **opportunity**?

Opportunities are around you each and everyday. Make a list of all your friends and colleagues and start enjoying a good meal with each of them. Remember to listen and forget about yourself. Write down at least ten people on a sheet of paper, pick up the phone, and have a cup of coffee with them. Two dollars at your local coffee shop–that's all it takes. The opportunities are endless.

What does **persistence** mean to me?

Persistence is the ability to face defeat again and again and again and again without giving up. I thank every inventor every day of my life. Thank goodness for electricity, phones, refrigerators, automobiles, airplanes, computers, and technology in general. That is persistence.

"What this power is I cannot say; all I know is that it exists and it becomes available only when a man is in the state of mind in which he knows exactly what he wants and is fully determined not to quit until he finds it." –ALEXANDER GRAHAM BELL

"If at first you don't succeed, try, try again." –WILLIAM E. HICKSON

POWERFUL QUESTIONS TO HELP YOU
MOVE FORWARD IN YOUR LIFE

How are you **persistent**?

What can you do to accomplish your goals? This truly is a key to your success. Don't worry about failure; just forge ahead. What are you willing to do to become successful?

How do I **plan** out my life?

Where am I today, and where am I going? If I want to achieve things in my life, I must have a plan. Planning is my map for getting to where I want to be.

I always write a plan, than I read my plan, I adjust my plan, and I always rewrite my plan. I make it simple, I make it complete, I make it my own.

"Developing the plan is actually laying out the sequence of events that have to occur for you to achieve your goal." –GEORGE L. MORRISEY

Begin today and map out what is ahead of you. Make a **plan**.

There are many books out there that can teach you how to design your plan, or just create your own. This page is blank. Start writing a plan.

What are my **possibilities**?

This is probably the easiest and toughest question I ask of myself or anyone. Most of us don't realize what is in front of us. Remember, there are truly no limits to the possibilities you have, and the number of possibilities is enormous. When you realize this, you truly start living your life.

We truly have more potential than we can ever develop in our lifetime. There is no limit to the possibilities. The unfortunate thing is that sometimes we put up a stop sign. We really don't know what we can do until we try.

My possibilities: I can write a book. I can give more of myself. I can do a triathlon. I can take more time for myself. I can spend more time with my family. I can be happier. Etc.

"We all have possibilities we don't know about. We can do things we don't even dream we can do." –DALE CARNEGIE

What are your **possibilities**?

There are so many. Just start with a few, and many will follow. No one is stopping you but you. When you finally understand this concept, it will be a day of awakening for you.

I am about to give you a gift of a lifetime. I am a superhero, and I can give you **the power to succeed**.

Close your eyes. Yes, please close them. But I guess you need to read this first.

Imagine I am standing next to you. I am a superhero with tremendous powers. I tap you on the shoulder and tell you, "I just gave you the power to control your own destiny!" How does this make you feel?

Start reading books and educate yourself because you have the power to do what you want to do. It's that simple.

"Knowledge is power." –THOMAS HOBBES

POWERFUL QUESTIONS TO HELP YOU
MOVE FORWARD IN YOUR LIFE

What is your **destiny**?

You have the power to control it. Now go out and get it. What do you truly want out of life?

Who am I **responsible** for?

I have responsibility to my family, to society, to my faith, and most of all, to myself. I am responsible for my success, and I am absolutely responsible for my failures. I am responsible for my own actions. When you stop taking responsibility for your actions, you have no control.

My father once told me, "We come into this world naked with nothing but the hope of love from our parents, and some don't even receive that. We leave this world stripped down with no one else lying beside us. We need to be responsible for our own actions, our own desires, and our own knowledge. No one controls us but us."
–GENE GARLIN

I miss you, Dad!

What does **responsibility** mean to you?

List your current responsibilities; we all have them. What kind of picture do you have right now of yourself? Life is not easy, but how you manage your responsibilities can be changed for the better. I know you can do it. I know you can make your life better.

What does **success** mean to me?

Success to me is doing the best I can each and every day and moving forward in my life. Success is a personal statement that only each individual can answer alone.

Is success learning how to ride a bike, or is success actually trying to ride a bike? If you want to change your health, then just start walking, drinking water, and eating fruits and vegetables. You are now succeeding.

"I do the very best I know how—the very best I can; and I mean to keep on doing so until the end." —ABRAHAM LINCOLN

What does **success** mean to you?

Do I tell the **truth**? If I don't, why not?

Truth is reality. Don't hide it; share it. When I lead a life of truth, it can be difficult at times, but wow, what a difference it makes.

If I do one thing in life, I will always be truthful!

I have seen this over and over again, not being truthful can shorten your life. Stress, anxiety, and feeling ill all comes from not being truthful to yourself and to others.

"Everything has its way of working out in the end. Truth just makes it happen quicker." –ANONYMOUS

POWERFUL QUESTIONS TO HELP YOU
MOVE FORWARD IN YOUR LIFE

Do you tell the **truth**? If not, why?

POWERFUL QUESTIONS TO HELP YOU
MOVE FORWARD IN YOUR LIFE

What is my **vision**?

The more we see, the more we can achieve. The courage to follow our dreams, our passions, our life as we see it—this must be our vision.

My vision is helping others through my work and spending time with the people whom I love and care about. It's a big vision, and I live it every day.

"The most pathetic person in the world is some one who has sight but no vision." –HELEN KELLER

What is your **vision**?

ABOUT THE AUTHOR

Michael Garlin is a father, husband, brother, son, friend, and teacher. Michael's passion in life is to laugh, smile, and live by the philosophy that one must give without ever expecting to get something back.

Michael's education:
School of Hard Knocks: Don't we all graduate from here?
Arizona State University: Bachelor of Science Recreation
Nova University: Master of Science Human Services
Coaches Training Institute: Certified Professional Co-Active Coach (CPCC)

I learn every day from everyone who surrounds me.

Read every day; that is the best education you can ever receive.

For those who are interested in Michael's services as a motivational speaker (get ready to think & laugh) or healthy life coach (get ready to change your life), you must think of yourself or your organization as being ready to move forward. Are you ready to get healthy? Do you have gaps to fill, and are you ready for the tough questions? Are you ready to make a difference?

Contact Michael Garlin:

www.iamstartingonmonday.com

michael@iamstartingonmonday.com

This book was written with you in mind. Enjoy.

www.ingramcontent.com/pod-product-compliance
Lightning Source LLC
Chambersburg PA
CBHW060518290526
45791CB00001B/441